What
I've Learned
About Sex

What I've Learned About *Sex*

Leading Sex Educators, Therapists, and Researchers Share Their Secrets

DEBRA W. HAFFNER, MPH, *and*
PEPPER SCHWARTZ, Ph.D.

A PERIGEE BOOK

A Perigee Book
Published by The Berkley Publishing Group
A member of Penguin Putnam Inc.
200 Madison Avenue
New York, NY 10016

First edition: October 1998

Published simultaneously in Canada.

The Penguin Putnam Inc. World Wide Web site address is
http://www.penguinputnam.com

Library of Congress Cataloging-in-Publication Data
Haffner, Debra.
    What I've learned about sex : leading sex educators,
therapists, and researchers share their secrets / Debra W. Haffner
and Pepper Schwartz. — 1st ed.
        p.   cm.
    "A Perigee book."
    Includes bibliographical references.
    ISBN 0-399-52439-8
    1. Sex—Miscellanea. 2. Sex customs—Miscellanea.
3. Man-woman relationships—Miscellanea.
4. Sexologists—Quotations.
I. Schwartz, Pepper. II. Title.
HQ21.H26   1998
306.7—dc21   98-6086
                                                             CIP

Printed in the United States of America

10   9   8   7   6   5   4   3   2   1

Contents

Contents

Contributors

We are grateful to the following professionals for contributing their thoughts for this volume: John Bancroft, Kathryn N. Black, Diane Brashear, Peggy Brick, Gila Bronner, Vern L. Bullough, Vivienne Cass, Eli Coleman, Al Cooper, Janice Epp, Helen Fisher, Marilyn Fithian, Sol Gordon, Kathryn Hanley, Elaine Hatfield, Sharon Kerr, Marty Klein, Robert Kolodny, Janet Lever, Amy Levine, Jim Maddock, Neil McConaghy, Charles Moser, Charlene Muehlenhard, Peter Naus, Gina Ogden, Carolyn Patierno,

Richard C. Pillard, Wardell Pomeroy, Domeena C. Renshaw, Ray Rosen, Marilyn Safir, Robert Selverstone, Peter Sandor Gardos, Judy Seifer, Brian Spitzberg, Susan Sprecher, William R. Stayton, Leonore Tiefer, Roy Bowen Ward, Jodi Wallace, David L. Weis, Susan Wilson, Beverly Whipple, William Yarber, and Yuriy Zharkov.

Introduction

This book was born over a lengthy breakfast. We are sexologists by profession, and good friends. It's only natural that our conversations often turn to sexuality issues. While talking about the impact of our work on our own personal lives and decisions, we were struck by how much our own lives are enhanced by our professional knowledge and experiences.

Fortunately, our jobs have given us a unique education in sexuality. Yet, most Americans have had little sexuality education as teenagers in school, and less as adults. Most people have few places, and few people, to turn to for information, other than their doctors or popular magazines.

As sexologists, we have reaped the benefits of years of professional training, study, and research. We have had the chance to examine our own attitudes and beliefs about sexuality with other professionals. Perhaps most important, we also have had the privilege and the honor to talk with hundreds, sometimes thousands, of people each year about their sexual experiences, questions, and concerns.

We realized that we wanted to share what we've learned with others, and knew that our colleagues felt the same way. But too often, our insights are buried in research articles or 600-page books that few have the time or inclination to read.

We decided to ask other sexologists for their best insights, expressed in the most accessible terms. In one or two sentences, we wanted these experts to relate the most important things they've learned about sex and sexuality over the years. We sent a letter to colleagues who are members of the three major sexological associations in the U.S.: the Sexuality Information and Education Council of the United States, the American Association of Sex Educators, Counselors, and Therapists, and the Society for the Scientific Study of Sexuality. The response was gratifying.

The resulting compilation is based on the belief that sexuality is much more than sex, or physical acts and the biology of reproduction. Sexuality also includes our attitudes, beliefs, and values about identity, relationships, and intimacy. It is about who we are as men and women, and how we relate to each other—not just about what we do in bed. The chapters in this book address sexuality in its broadest definition, and include information about relationships, body image, identity, sexual health, sexual behaviors, and sexuality and culture.

This book is also based on our belief that information empowers people to make the best decisions about their own sexuality and sexual lives. We believe that moral, responsible sexual relationships are consensual, non-exploitative, honest, mutually pleasurable, and protected against disease and unwanted pregnancy.

We've compiled this material in order to provide mini-lessons on sexuality. Glance at a few entries a day, or read the book from cover to cover. Whatever your method, we hope that this book educates you, reassures you, and amuses you. The vast majority of sexologists would embrace many of the statements included within these pages.

Other entries are more controversial and represent the contributor's personal ideas and experiences. Of course, not every insight rings true for every individual. Some of the entries offer practical advice; others will make you think more about your own attitudes and experiences. We hope that you will share some of them with your friends, partners, and families.

This book is for ADULTS. We assume that you have had some sexual experience, and we hope that you have a sense of humor. And although this is not a "how to" book, we hope it will give you ideas and information to help you celebrate your sexuality.

Please keep in mind that this book is not a substitute for individual counseling and medical advice. In the last chapter of the book, you'll find a list of organizations, hotline numbers, and Internet addresses to refer to for more in-depth information and help.

We've also learned more about sexuality as we compiled and edited these entries. While working together, we learned anew that sexuality education is a lifelong process, and a central part of who we are. Perhaps most importantly, we were reminded again that there is always more to learn about this wonderful, vital part of our lives.

About SEX

I've learned that...

Having sex and making love are rarely the same.

"Going through the motions" is almost never worth it.

Sex and sexuality are two different things. Sex is what you do with your body; sexuality is who you are.

Sex is not the same thing as intercourse.

Married couples should spend as much time thinking about what they are going to do in bed on the weekend as they do thinking about where they are going with their friends.

I've learned that...

When a person is acting by choice, sex is the most ecstatic celebration of body and spirit; when it's not by choice, sex is an extreme violation of body and spirit.

Sex can be just as much fun now as it was when I was 18.

Sex is for you. Have it for yourself and not for someone else. But if you do decide to have it for someone else, make sure it's also right for you.

Sex is a small part of life, but it becomes very important when it doesn't work out.

Sex is fun. If it isn't fun, you're on the wrong track.

Sexuality is a matter of invention and choice.

It is a myth that sex just comes naturally; people need to learn to be good lovers.

Most cultures convey negative messages about sexuality; we have to work to appreciate our sexuality and celebrate it.

What I've Learned About Sex

I've learned that...

There are some things that can only be expressed through sex.

Sex is wonderful! You don't have to feel guilty to enjoy it.

The principal value of sex is its potential for fostering intimacy between two people.

Even though sex can be very special, people get in trouble by expecting far too much from it or from themselves.

The vulnerability we show during sex is a powerful way to build trust and intimacy.

People are surprisingly willing to settle for a mediocre sex life instead of taking concrete steps to change it.

I can enjoy sexual feelings about another person and not act on them.

We are both sexual and spiritual beings. One of our major tasks in life is to integrate these. I've learned that too often organized religion has split our sexual and spiritual selves.

I've learned that. . .

All sexual decisions have consequences of some kind.

Both men and women can experience sexual pleasure throughout their lives.

People with disabilities have the same need for intimacy and sexuality as people without disabilities.

Decisions about sexual relationships continue throughout life.

Having a good—even a great—sex life does not guarantee happiness . . . but it helps.

Thinking before sex is a good idea; thinking during sex never is.

America is one of the most sexually ambivalent cultures in the world.

There are more than 70,000 Web pages containing the word *sex*.

Sex is the most commonly searched topic on the Internet.

What I've Learned About Sex

I've learned that. . .

Americans are so worried about sexuality that half of the states uphold laws prohibiting certain types of sexual behaviors between consenting adults.

In the 1990s, people have intercourse at earlier ages and marry later.

Sex is a whole-person proposition: body, mind, heart, and soul.

Sexual energy gets charged way before you enter the bedroom, and if the relationship is good, it lasts long afterwards.

In some states, it's legal to buy a gun, but not a vibrator.

Millions of years of evolution have given us the opportunity to enjoy sex.

With sex, as with so many other things, someone else's grass is not always greener.

Men and women can be attracted to each other, yet remain friends without becoming physically involved—but only if they can talk about it.

$\mathcal{I}'$ve learned that...

You'll always remember your first time.

One of the ways to kill a good sex life is to have a TV in the bedroom.

All people are sexual even if they never have sex with another person.

2

About
MEN

I've learned that. . .

Men want reassurance after the baby arrives. Tired as you both may be, take time to have a great experience in bed before too much time elapses.

You shouldn't tell men anything about other lovers you had before them. The jealous ones will get nasty. The non-jealous ones will think you are tacky.

Some men truly prefer some extra weight on a woman. Assume they do, and they probably will.

I've learned that...

Men love fantasy stories. Meet in a bar and pretend you are two people getting turned on to each other for the first time.

Sometimes men want rough and tumble, physically aggressive sex.

Men think it's great when women are really unself-conscious and forget about their hair, their clothes, and lose themselves in the heat of the moment.

Some men really like having their prostate stroked—and some men hate it. Experiment and ask.

Only a few men really care about breast size.

If a man does really care about breast size, avoid him.

Even a conservative man will like sexy clothes—when they are worn only for him. Or ordinary clothes worn with no underwear.

Covert sexual touching in public places drives some men crazy.

What I've Learned About Sex

I've learned that...

If men bought as many "how to" books on sex as they buy books about golf and tennis, they would have more sex.

All men—at one time or another—have a difficult time getting an erection.

Men who can't get erections routinely often have physical, not psychological, problems.

A surprising number of younger men have erectile problems; the mean age for beginning urinary and erectile problems is 37.

There are many new treatments for male erectile problems; more men ought to see their friendly neighborhood urologist.

Too many men are now relying on new technologies (like pills and injections) to achieve erections—rather than learning about their feelings.

I've learned that...

Many men hate condoms so much that they will pay a prostitute extra not to wear one. If they feel strongly about not wearing one with you, they probably have been exactly the same way with someone else—perhaps recently.

Variety is the road to a man's sexual interest. If you normally make love on the bed, try making love someplace else. Don't miss a room in your house.

Most men, on most occasions, do not want "just sex" from a partner; like women, they want affection, closeness and affirmation.

Too many men think the only way they can get closeness and affection is through genital sex.

Most men really do want to feel that they hold the key to their partner's ecstasy. But some men get scared when a woman is really out of control. The trick is knowing what kind of man you have.

Sometimes all a man wants is a quickie . . . but that doesn't mean he doesn't care about you.

Men like women to initiate sex—but not more often than they do.

I've learned that...

Most men really want to go to sleep after sex—let them.

Showering and scented soaps or creams can make a difference in how a man feels about oral sex.

Putting on a condom can feel sexy or sleazy—it all depends on how it's done. Take it slowly; make it a sensual part of the seduction process.

Many men like to have their nipples caressed.

New sexual acts should be introduced gradually; an overly quick introduction might make him feel embarrassed.

More men should understand that giving sexy lingerie every so often is a good idea.

Some men find flannel sexier than lace. Experiment and see whether he likes you more in satin—or his shirt.

Only about one in six men have ever paid for sex.

Men are turned on by happy women.

$\mathcal{I}$'ve learned that...

Every man should have a weekend alone with his long-term partner at least once every three months.

If you are an oral sex artist, chances are you will own his soul.

If you lubricate a lot, let him feel it. It's a vote of confidence from your body that will excite him.

Men like a frank show of interest, but let them win you over.

Men are more confused about sex now than ever before.

Most men have difficulty accepting that erections are not a matter of will.

Some men like you to use a vibrator on them.

Good oral sex is much more than putting a penis in a mouth; using the tongue under the head of the penis, down the shaft, and on the scrotum makes it special.

Men want a woman who can be a good mother—but not in bed.

I've learned that...

It's best not to think or speak about children right before you make love.

Dancing with a man who really dances well is very effective foreplay.

3

About WOMEN

<u>*I've learned that. . .*</u>
A woman wants a man who takes the time to learn about her body and desires, not one who makes her feel that he makes love this way with everyone.

Women are not shy or coy about displaying sexual interest in a man. When a woman wants sex with a particular man, she sends unmistakable signals.

When a woman appears uninterested, she is.

Most women want great reactions, obvious delight, and flattering remarks—but no lines—about their bodies.

I've learned that. . .

You can never say too many nice things to a woman during sex—as long as you mean them.

Generic endearments, like "Oh Baby," are a big turn-off.

Some people still don't know that the vagina isn't the same as a penis; for almost all women, it's the clitoris that is the source of greatest sexual pleasure.

Women get really upset if you promise one single thing you don't follow through on.

An advantage of female sexuality is that arousal and orgasm can occur in a public place without anyone knowing.

A woman wants to know if a new lover has trouble maintaining an erection. If she knows, she will feel nurturing, helpful. If it just happens, she will take it personally, and be hurt, angry, or disappointed.

A really quick ejaculation is almost never taken as a compliment. It can be passed off as one—but only once.

I've learned that...

A man who really takes time touching a woman—her ears, her throat, the backs of her knees, her toes—is truly sexy and truly appreciated.

A man who is good at bringing home lingerie is suspect.

Women will say they want to know if there is anyone else. They do. But if you tell them there is, it will ruin everything.

It may look or feel great to plunge deeply into a woman— but it can also be painful. Work up to going in deeply. Make sure it's what she wants.

A man should keep asking—make it easy for her to tell you what she needs.

If you're uncertain, use a light touch. Let her tell you if it should be more forceful.

Good sex can happen without a penis.

I've learned that...

Using your eyes to convey your belief that your partner is the most desirable woman in the universe is the sexiest, most intimate thing you can do during sex.

A man who has obviously prepared for sex by being clean and smelling sweet has already begun foreplay.

Women love to be asked, "What would you like me to do?"—but not right away. Passion and tenderness are more important than technique—at least in the beginning.

Women want men who are sensitive enough to keep their fingernails clean and short.

Men who look at other women when you are with them are insensitive and callous. Don't show a woman that she doesn't hold your complete attention.

A man who takes off your clothes slowly and with great intensity and pleasure is a sexy man.

One of the sexiest feelings in the world is the feeling of a man in jeans, so close to you that you can feel his erection through the material.

I've learned that...

Really fragrant flowers brought to the bedroom on a special night can help set the mood.

Most women get extremely aroused making love spontaneously in the kitchen or living room.

Some of the sexiest things you can do with a woman are stroking her hair, lightly touching her face, and tracing her eyes, nose and mouth.

Some women also like to fall asleep right after orgasm.

It's very arousing if you make sure you touch every part of her during sex: the vagina, the inside, the lips, and the clitoris.

It's important to apply a good lubricant if necessary; saliva doesn't work well, and petroleum jelly destroys condoms.

The way to a woman's heart is by soft kisses.

The jackhammer approach to the clitoris almost never works.

I've learned that...

Staying awake after orgasm—at least for a little while—matters to most women.

It's best not to ask a woman, "Did you come?"

Slowly, tenderly washing a woman's hair is very erotic.

If women knew as much about sex as they do about diets, they would be happier.

Kegel exercises really do a) increase the strength of your vaginal muscles, b) increase your bladder control, and c) make intercourse more pleasurable for you and your partner.

Women can almost always tell if their sexual partner is thinking about something else.

I don't have to be a sex goddess; being good is good enough.

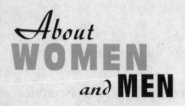

4

About
WOMEN
and MEN

I've learned that...

Men and women differ more when it comes to sex than gays and straights.

Women still wait by the phone more than men do.

If a man walks by a window where a woman is undressing and looks in, he is a voyeur; if a woman walks by a window where a man is undressing and looks in, he is an exhibitionist.

The double standard about sex still exists.

Men also can fake orgasms.

I've learned that...

Most women don't have orgasms through intercourse alone.

Most women love oral sex—and most men haven't learned to do it well.

Most men love oral sex—and most women haven't learned to do it well.

Even in liberated couples, the men still take out the garbage and the women buy the children's clothes.

Straight men are more threatened by homosexuality than straight women are.

Almost a quarter of all women say that they've ever been forced to have sex—but only 3 percent of men say that they've ever forced anyone to have sex.

Teenage girls are more likely to wish that they had waited to have intercourse than teenage boys.

I've learned that...

There are still people who think that women who carry condoms on first dates are sluts—and that men are just prepared.

Most men really don't like using condoms—and to most women, they really don't make a difference.

Most men still leave contraception up to their partners.

Both men and women like sexually explicit videos—just not always the same ones.

Men usually have more sexual partners in their lifetimes than women, but not by a lot.

Women need more support to say "yes" and men need more support to say "no."

Women who love sex are too often called "sluts" or "promiscuous," and men who love sex are called "studs."

One in three women say they just aren't interested in sex, but only one in six men admit that they aren't interested.

I've learned that...

More than half of men but only one in five women say that they think about sex every day or several times a day.

Men are more likely to be uninhibited about sex than women—but not always.

Men want more sex when they're younger, and women want more sex when they're older. Maybe more younger men and older women should be together.

There are more men than women who would like to have impersonal sex.

Men have more performance anxiety than women.

Even the most liberated men and women sometimes want to be treated traditionally.

Most men consider their wives to be their best friends; most women turn to other women for friendship.

I've learned that...

Women want their children sleeping in the marital bed more than their spouses do.

Women read a whole lot more books on sex than men do; it's that being lost and asking for directions thing.

Men and women are more alike than different.

5

About ATTRACTION

I've learned that...

Lust and love are different, but it's easy to confuse the two at first.

Every pot has a cover. Everyone will be attracted to someone.

Opposites do attract, but it's easier to have a long-term relationship with someone similar to yourself—at least in important ways.

Most people are usually attracted to one particular physical type.

I've learned that...

People can get more attractive as they age—but only if they work at it.

More people have same-sex attractions than act upon them.

Some people seem to always be attracted to people who aren't good for them.

Beauty really is in the eye of the beholder.

As a straight man, a flirtatious comment from a gay man is a compliment rather than a threat to my masculinity.

Some people are first attracted to eyes . . . faces . . . breasts . . . hands . . . feet . . . forearms . . . buttocks . . . Any part of the body can be someone's turn-on.

People would be better off if they understood that they can feel sexually attracted to someone without necessarily acting on it . . . or even commenting on it.

Sometimes I will be attracted to people who have no interest in me . . . and vice versa.

$\mathcal{I}$'ve learned that...

It's often better not to tell someone you are attracted to them . . . especially if you haven't gotten any clues that they are attracted to you.

People in couples are still attracted to other people . . . and they have to continually choose not to act on their feelings.

Not everyone is attracted to model-perfect bodies.

If I'm feeling attractive, I'm more likely to be attractive to someone else.

I can get aroused just by smelling the perfume of someone I love.

People are usually attracted to people who are clearly attracted to them.

When there's chemistry, you have to choose whether to acknowledge it.

Locking eyes with someone for the first time can be a very sexy moment.

I've learned that...

When people are open to being attractive to others, they have a special aura.

A lot of middle-class women are intensely attracted to working-class men, but they almost never marry them.

Physical attraction is a poor foundation for a long-term relationship, but some physical attraction is essential.

Being outgoing and feeling good about yourself makes you more attractive than a model-like face and body.

People who have just fallen in love have a special glow.

What I wear has a great deal to do with how attractive I feel.

Part of what makes a man or woman attractive is a certain sexual self-confidence that makes you feel they will be great in bed.

A woman without makeup has her own special attractive-ness.

As I get older, I look worse when I wake up.

I've learned that...

Many men find a pregnant woman especially attractive.

Most people are very uncomfortable and embarrassed when you tell them how attractive they are.

Men and women who feel good about their bodies are more attractive to others.

6

About BODIES

I've learned that...
A key to good sex is liking and knowing your own body.

While there are differences in flaccid penis size, once erect most penises appear pretty much the same. Some men are "show-ers" and some men are "grow-ers."

There are small penises and big penises, and women have different opinions about which feel better.

In the United States, some women have problems with uncircumcised penises, but not after they fall in love with men who have them.

I've learned that. . .

Vulvas vary in appearance from one woman to another.

Penises look quite different from one another.

I can appreciate the beauty of both male and female genitals.

Few people look like the media ideal—and it doesn't really matter.

A majority of American women—and increasing numbers of American men—are unhappy with their bodies.

A sexy slip or nightgown can do wonders for your body image.

Most bodies look the same lying down.

Men are more concerned about penis size than women are.

I will never look as good as I did at 18 . . . but I'm a much better lover.

I've learned that...

Many women have one breast that is larger than the other . . . sometimes a cup size or more.

People with the best bodies are usually not the best lovers.

Having babies doesn't help your body image.

As I've gotten older, personality turns me on more than physical perfection.

Some women feel sexiest when they are pregnant.

Most American women are on a diet, coming off a diet, or thinking about going on a diet.

Many people prefer to make love with the lights off because they are disappointed with their bodies.

A good lover makes me feel beautiful.

A majority of people say they like watching their partners undress.

Feeling comfortable with your own nude body makes you a better lover.

I've learned that...

Men tend to be most self-conscious about their chests and women tend to worry most about their hips and thighs.

Many women want to be thinner than men want them to be.

More and more men are getting cosmetic surgery.

As they get older, even women who once considered wearing makeup a nonfeminist act are considering coloring their hair and having their eyes done.

Breast reduction or augmentation is a serious operation and should be considered very carefully.

Even people with perfect bodies think they are imperfect.

Different ethnic and racial communities have different standards of beauty.

The popularity of the Wonder Bra means that many women still think that sexiness is signified by big breasts and cleavage.

I've learned that. . .

Young men now feel much the same pressure as young women to be fit, toned, and sexy.

Most people don't have a realistic body image and are too hard on themselves.

7

About
COMMUNICATION

I've learned that...

It's better never to talk about how to improve our sex life after we've just had sex.

Many people lie about their sexual histories.

It is hard to be honest about past sexual experiences with a new partner.

Some sexual secrets—unless they pose a health threat—are better left unshared.

Nonverbal communication often works better than words in bed.

I've learned that...

Even sexologists can have a difficult time communicating about sexual needs, limits, and desires with a partner.

Many people think that planning for sex—and talking about it beforehand—may make it less likely to happen.

Couples can talk themselves out of having sex.

Talking during sex—sharing fantasies, using forbidden words—can be very sexy.

Many men have pet names for their penises and like you to use them.

Sometimes you need to see a counselor in order to talk about sexual problems.

It's better not to ask my partner, "What are you thinking?" when he's just being quiet.

Couples who have nothing to say to each other in restaurants are usually married—and they may be in trouble.

I've learned that...

Open, honest communication is the most important foundation for a relationship.

Sometimes "he just doesn't understand me" is the truth—and I have to accept it.

You cannot underestimate the value of humor.

After humor, consideration is the second most important ingredient in a sexual relationship. Most people appreciate a sensitive and thoughtful partner. To quote a song, "It's the little things that matter most."

Communicating what you like to a partner is easier than communicating what you don't like.

Most people aren't comfortable talking about sexual issues.

It's hard to know if someone is really being honest with you about their past sexual experiences or their current motives.

Consent requires communication.

I've learned that...

"Yes" doesn't always mean "yes," and "no" doesn't always mean "no." "No" really does sometimes mean "maybe", but I still need to be sure that my partner is truly consenting.

In a new sexual relationship, it is better to ask than assume consent.

It is fear of rejection that can make honest communication so difficult.

Many people seem to have difficulty expressing their desire for sex in words. We should be able to do better; after all, we don't rub up against the refrigerator to show we are hungry.

It's better to talk about sexual feelings, desires and boundaries in relationships.

It is hard to negotiate sexual limits and behaviors with a new partner—and even harder with a long-term partner.

Talking about sex is sometimes better than doing it.

What I've Learned About Sex

I've learned that...

Talking seriously about sex over the telephone is hard to do and probably should wait until two people are together.

Older people often find it just as hard as young people to discuss sexual issues with their partners.

It is hard to know how to request something during lovemaking; some partners feel pressured or dominated, and others take any request as a criticism.

Talking about scenes in movies or books can sometimes be a good way to communicate what you like in sex and relationships.

The key to great sex is being able to communicate exactly what you want in a way your partner can hear and feel good about.

Talking during lovemaking makes the experience more intimate.

8

About
CONTRACEPTION
and CONDOMS

I've learned that...

There still isn't a contraceptive method that's 100 percent effective, 100 percent safe, and 100 percent sexy.

Using the pill makes some women more interested in sex, and others less interested.

Research shows that using a condom is 10,000 times safer than not using one.

Occasionally condoms do break; make sure you leave room at the tip and that there is plenty of lubrication.

I've learned that. . .

The more practice you have with condoms, the less chance there is of breakage or slippage.

Hardly anyone really uses condoms and foam together— but they should.

Putting my diaphragm in before we start having sex cuts down on awkwardness.

You have to check your diaphragm for holes; older ones can get brittle and break.

You have to replace your diaphragm every few years.

Women need to have their diaphragms resized after the birth of a baby or after gaining or losing ten pounds, and I've learned this the hard way.

Once a guy knows a woman is on the pill, it's harder to get him to use a condom—but it's still necessary.

People who know better sometimes pick passion over safety.

IUDs are not a good choice if you have multiple partners.

I've learned that...

More women still opt to be sterilized even though it's safer for men.

You need to use contraception at least a year past menopause.

It's safe for women over 40 to be on the pill, unless they are smokers.

Low-dose oral contraceptives can be a boon to women in the years right before menopause.

There are many types of condoms. If you don't like one brand, keep trying until you find one that's pleasurable.

It's fun to use colored condoms.

Flavored condoms taste terrible; who are they kidding?

The contraceptive jelly goes in after oral sex.

It's a mistake to keep the contraceptive jelly next to my toothpaste.

Getting sterilized can boost your sex life.

I've learned that...

Condoms make men last longer and that can make them better lovers.

Having a lover put the condom on—or the diaphragm in—can be very sexy.

Some men lose their erections while putting on condoms. Practice alone usually solves the problem.

Most men leave contraception up to the woman.

Most contraceptive failures happen because people don't use them correctly—or at all.

Only condoms reliably prevent most sexually transmitted diseases.

Condoms do not always prevent the transmission of genital warts.

Both women and men should carry condoms.

Even as an adult, I find it embarrassing to buy condoms at my local drugstore.

I've learned that...

A woman should go to a physician who specializes in Norplant if that's the kind of contraception she wants.

People will ask, "What's that thing in your arm?" if you're using Norplant. You have to decide in advance how you'll answer that question.

Sometimes my diaphragm still flies across the room.

For people who don't want to deal with contraception, Depo Provera is a good temporary method.

No matter how well you think you know your partner, if you both don't know your HIV status AND you're not 100 percent sure that your partner is completely monogamous, you should always use a condom.

Most men will not insist on using a condom even when they ought to.

A man doesn't need to know that I'm having my period if I wear a diaphragm.

Now more than ever you need to think about BOTH preventing pregnancies and protecting yourself against STDs.

You can be both spontaneous and responsible.

9

About
DATING

I've learned that. . .

Having intercourse on the first date usually means there won't be a second date.

If you haven't had intercourse after dating for three months, then it's probably not going to happen.

If a person is not attracted to someone on the first date, they probably never will be.

There are surprising exceptions to the above generalizations.

$\mathcal{I}$'ve learned that...

The first time you kiss someone is one of the sweetest, most heart-pounding sexual experiences there is—no matter how old you are.

Men are supposed to be respectful on the first date, and try something by the third.

The more some men spend on a woman on a date, the more sex they expect.

"If you really love me, you'll have sex with me" is always a line.

Men who didn't date much when they were young are sweeter when they date as an adult.

Divorced men and women have sex sooner in a dating relationship than younger single men and women.

A big rich dinner can kill your desire for great sex that evening. And too much alcohol for men can hamper more than desire.

I've learned that...

Sex you regret happens frequently at fraternity parties and big alcoholic bashes.

Most men don't believe they are forcing a woman even when they are.

Too many men will try to at least argue with a woman when she says she doesn't want to have sex on a date.

When women dress like sex kittens on a date, it doesn't mean they are.

Many single men and women do not tell the truth about whether they have had a sexually transmitted disease.

Some single men and women do not know if they have had a sexually transmitted disease.

If a man says he loves you on the second or third date he thinks it entitles him to sex.

Whenever you have sex with a woman, no matter how short a time you have been dating, she needs to say how much she cares about you and she wants you to say the same.

I've learned that...

Most women who say they want to have sex on a date—no strings attached—are kidding themselves.

A surprising number of men cannot achieve or sustain an erection the first time you have intercourse with them.

Lesbians have sex on the first date a whole lot more often than I thought they would.

A lot more gay men do not have sex on the first date than I thought would.

The place where you have sex after a date is one of the most important factors that determine whether or not you enjoy the sexual experience.

It's hard to start dating again at 45.

My friends who are over 45 and who really want to get remarried, do.

Some people start going out with other people almost immediately after a breakup, while other people take years to begin dating again.

I've learned that...

If you want to date, you have to take risks and go where you might meet people.

I shouldn't bring my dates home to have sex when my kids are at home until I know that it is a committed relationship.

One of the nicer things about dating the second time around is that sex is not as urgent.

No matter how good the sex is, it's never worth being in a manipulative or exploitative relationship.

If you want to get married, think about meeting people through friends, or at school, work, a party, or church. That's where most people meet their spouses.

The Internet is a good way to meet others and practice dating skills, but you have to be very cautious about taking it "off-line."

"Dating" on-line can allow for pretty meaningful conversation. If you do meet, and you've both been honest, there can be a high level of intimacy.

I've learned that...

Ninety percent of Americans marry for the first time by the age of 30.

If a man is not sexually adventurous while you're dating, he's not going to be after you're married.

Getting married does not increase the frequency of a couple's sex life.

People are grateful if the person they are dating gets up in the morning and brushes his or her teeth before kissing or starting to make love.

Too many women find themselves in compromising and dangerous situations with men they don't know very well.

Some people stay married to avoid dating.

10

About
DESIRE
and SEXUAL ACTS

I've learned that...

Seduction is the first part of sexual response.

Many couples are not well matched when it comes to desire.

Many engaged couples knew they were not sexually well matched, and got married anyway.

Disorders of desire are the most frequent sexual problem . . . and often the hardest to treat.

It is not always the man who wants sex more frequently.

$\mathcal{I}$'ve learned that...

I prefer the excitement phase to last as long as possible.

Nothing builds desire like a long-term friendship slowly becoming sexual.

For almost all men it takes longer for them to get an erection as they age . . . and more time for them to want to have sex again . . . unless it's with a new lover.

Research tells us that one in ten adult women and one in three men have more than ten sexual partners in their lifetimes. Today's younger people are having more lovers earlier, and will probably have more partners in their lifetimes.

Some women's orgasms are stronger and quicker on a full bladder.

Women with cystitis shouldn't try for a strong, quick orgasm on a full bladder.

Even though it's not currently politically correct, there is really nothing like the pleasure of the first night with a new partner.

I've learned that...

People have the most sex partners when they are in their twenties.

For most people sex lasts for fifteen to twenty minutes, from kissing to orgasm to sleeping.

Both men and women prefer receiving oral sex to giving it.

One in four heterosexuals has had anal sex, and one in ten did so in the past year.

People may not tell the truth to sex researchers.

Sometimes it's worth trying to see if you can become aroused, even if you start out thinking that you are not interested.

Sometimes holding hands in a darkened movie theater can be more arousing than what follows.

Sex is like chocolate—the more you have, the more you want.

The most important sexual organs are the brain and the skin, not the genitals.

I've learned that...

Having sex when you are under pressure to perform is like being on the first golf tee with everyone watching.

What turns people on is not predictable and differs from one person to another.

If you don't tell an adolescent girl about her clitoris— where it is and what it's for—she'll think she's in love with the first boy who finds it.

Nearly three-quarters of both married and single adults had one sex partner last year.

People should take care that their sexual desire does not overwhelm their better judgment about what is important in life.

It is possible to have really great sex with a partner without having intercourse.

You should take off your eyeglasses when having oral sex.

I've learned that...

It's best not to scream during sex when there are thin walls and people are in the house—if I don't want people to break in and rescue me.

A new attractive partner can do wonders for someone who thinks they have low sexual desire.

Spouses who deeply desire one another are usually very happy people.

There are three responses to a sexual invitation: 1) "Yes, I'd like to"; 2) "No, I don't want to"; and 3) "I'm not particularly interested, but I'm willing if you are."

The more powerful a woman is in her relationship, the more likely she is to use the woman-on-top position.

It's hard to have sex standing up unless the two partners are about the same height.

If a partner doesn't like oral sex, it's hard to change his or her mind.

When I'm really turned on, it's sometimes hard to tell pain from pleasure.

The major ingredient of desire is being desired.

11

About
EXTRAMARITAL
SEX

I've learned that...

People should only have an affair if they can do it without fear or guilt.

Some affairs break up marriages and others keep them together.

It's best never to tell.

Unless you want to break up your marriage, only have an affair with someone who has as much to lose as you do.

Most affairs don't turn into lifelong relationships.

I've learned that...

Affairs always involve some risk.

Scrupulous STD and pregnancy prevention are critical for people having affairs.

I should never give out my home phone number or address.

Married men and women often treat their lovers better than their own spouses.

If your partner suddenly starts doing something new in bed, he probably learned it somewhere else.

The discovery of an affair will always cause a crisis in a marriage.

E-mail and voice mail aren't always private.

Your partner's credit card bill may be the most eloquent piece of information you have about whether or not he or she is having an affair.

The answer to "Are you having an affair?" is always "No."

I've learned that...

A partner who doesn't want you to act spontaneously—such as changing your plans to join him on a business trip—has something to hide.

The criteria for deciding whether or not to start an affair with someone must include belief in their character and integrity.

The safest affairs take place between people who live in different areas and work in different places.

People in good marriages have affairs.

People can't predict how an affair will affect them.

Adjoining hotel rooms help with discretion.

Having affairs can be expensive.

A noticeable change in sexual frequency—either less or more—could mean that your partner is having an affair.

Open marriages really don't work.

I've learned that...

At least three-quarters of all married people tell researchers that they have always been monogamous.

The "chase" for a new partner other than your spouse is often far more important than any subsequent sexual activity.

There is a big difference between an affair and a one-night stand.

Some people set themselves up to be caught.

Women should be suspicious if their husbands go out and buy themselves all new sexy underwear.

I should throw out any incriminating evidence before I go home.

If you have to keep a picture of your mistress, make sure it's a shot of her with her husband and children.

Marriages can survive after a spouse discovers an affair—but it usually takes professional help.

I've learned that...

If sex is missing from a marriage or not very fulfilling, there is a good chance that at least one of the partners will start having an affair.

After a partner finds out about an affair, there's a high risk that he or she will start one too.

Most women don't think that THEIR partner could ever have an affair. It's even more true for men.

Your children should NEVER know if you have ever had an affair.

Even your best friend shouldn't know about your affair.

Sometimes a person you've had an affair with can turn vindictive.

You really need to let your doctor know if you've had an affair since your last checkup.

Even affairs that seem totally safe can get emotionally out of hand.

I try to omit information as long as possible, and then I lie.

I've learned that...

An affair can make me feel sexy, desirable, and alive.

An affair can mean having just one more demanding person in your life.

Both men and women report that once a new potential partner agrees to be sexually intimate with them, most of the satisfaction has already been achieved.

More people considering an affair should say, "Thank you, that would have been lovely."

Many people don't have affairs for the sex; they can stroke their own genitals. The exhilaration comes from having someone new stroke their egos.

12

About FANTASY *and* SEXUALLY EXPLICIT MATERIALS

I've learned that...

People's fantasies are much wilder than I ever expected.

The most conventional person may have exotic fantasies and odd sexual desires.

No matter how sexually conservative a man is, he may fantasize about two women making love to each other.

Some heterosexual women find thinking about women making love to other women (or watching it on film) sexually erotic.

I've learned that...

Most heterosexual men get anxious when they see sexually explicit movies that include male-male sexuality.

Sadomasochistic fantasies are very common.

There are an infinite number of things that people fantasize about: shoes, leather, trees, wild animals, you name it.

If you feel guilty about a fantasy, the fantasy will come up over and over again.

Women daydream more about romance, and men daydream more about sexual acts.

Sexually explicit materials are harmless for most people; the only people they incite to sexual violence are already seriously disturbed.

I feel a lot better about reading sexually explicit materials myself than finding them under my child's bed.

I've learned that...

Many women's sexual fantasies and their interest in erotica are wilder than they will admit to others, and even to themselves.

Many women will like sexually explicit materials if they are not denigrating to women.

Most X-rated movies watched in bed don't get watched for more than the first five minutes.

People who enjoy taking nude or sexual pictures or home videos should destroy them THAT night.

The more I fantasize about someone, the hotter it is if we actually get together.

People can have vivid and compelling sexual fantasies that never have to be acted out.

Actually acting out a safe part of a fantasy can be thrilling. Make sure you and your partner agree on the content and the limits beforehand.

I can pick up new sexual techniques from X-rated movies.

I've learned that...

It's often better not to tell your partner about your sexual fantasies.

It can be exciting to talk about fantasies in bed with someone, but it's important to know your partner's limits.

Some people really like to be told erotic stories during lovemaking.

Telling erotic stories over the telephone can be a great addition to your regular sex life, or a substitute when you can't see the other person.

People are turned on by different types of erotica.

A lot of the sex we see on TV and the movies is pure fantasy. Most people aren't having sex that hot, that often.

There are now feminists producing erotica specifically for women.

X-rated videos are the most frequently rented videos at neighborhood stores.

$\mathcal{I}$'ve learned that. . .

I should not keep my erotica in my nightstand, but somewhere my children can't find it.

A lot of people feel unnecessarily guilty about their fantasies.

Acting out fantasies can be exciting—but it's hard to stay "in character."

One person's erotica is another person's pornography.

13

About LOVE *and* ROMANCE

I've learned that...

When you think you are in love, even badly performed sex is still thrilling.

Looking into each other's eyes during sex is the most romantic thing on the planet.

A lot of people say they are in love so they can justify having sex.

A little romance gets me into bed a lot sooner than a lot of lust.

If a man thinks he is in love, it can make him so nervous that he can't perform intercourse.

$\mathcal{I}$'ve learned that...

The answer to the question "How do I know if I'm in love?" is "If you feel you're in love, you are." But I've also learned that there are two kinds of love: mature and immature. After a few months, you can always tell the difference.

Mature love is energizing, and immature love is exhausting. In a mature love experience, you are nice to the world; when it's immature, you tend to be cranky and mean.

One of the most romantic things a person can do is say "I love you" right after orgasm.

One of the most romantic things a person can say is "I don't want to make love to anyone but you anymore."

A romantic movie is a very effective form of foreplay.

One of the most romantic ways to have sex is to have a picnic in the woods, in a private place, a safe spot—without mosquitoes or sudden visitors.

I've learned that...

Loving yourself first improves your ability to love another person.

You can enjoy sex without falling in love.

Loving someone is incomparably more complicated than making love to someone.

Being in love is not enough to ensure a good relationship. Friendship, trust, shared tasks and pleasures, and a sense of humor are essential ingredients.

Making love with a new partner can be so arousing that your hormones can trick you into thinking you're in love.

It's just as important to like your partner as it is to love him/her.

I am a junkie for romance, not sex.

Sometimes I don't want romance, I want sex—pure and simple.

Believing that no one loves me is the worst feeling in the world.

I've learned that...

I can love someone I don't really like.

A thirteen-year-old can be deeply in love—it's real love even if it doesn't last.

It's best not to call this puppy love.

You never love anyone quite like the person you first fell in love with when you were 16.

If a friend of mine thinks he or she is in love, even if I think it's a disaster, nothing I say will change his or her mind.

"Adrenaline really does make the heart grow fonder"— people fall in love during war, during personal crises, at weddings and funerals.

Even when a couple feels their love is dead, love can come back.

A fireplace and a glass of champagne creates the perfect setting for romance.

Lust clouds my ability to see my lover objectively.

I've learned that...

It's just as easy to fall in love with a nice guy as with a bad boy.

Some men will never love any woman as much as they loved their mothers. And those of us raising sons need to be aware of this.

One of the most vulnerable acts of one's life is to fall in love.

Periodically I re-fall in love with my own spouse—and that's wonderful.

Lifelong love is never as simple as "happily ever after."

Love is a skill.

Not enough marriage and sex counselors talk about love with their clients.

Being in love is not enough of a reason to get married.

When I'm in love or when I'm breaking up with someone, the songs on the radio start to make sense.

14

About

MARRIAGE
and LONG-TERM
RELATIONSHIPS

I've learned that...

You really have to work at keeping sex a priority in long-term relationships.

The longer the relationship, the less frequent the sex.

Vacations alone together can do wonders.

On vacations, sex is NOT always better.

Expecting sex to be better on vacations can sometimes cause too much pressure, and then disappointments.

I've learned that...

For some lucky people, sex gets better every year.

It is good to try new things with a long-term partner.

Children are parents' main barrier to a good sex life.

Sex improves when the children are old enough to sleep at their friends' houses.

Lucky couples have bedrooms on different floors than their children.

Married people have sex more frequently than single people.

Married couples on average spend less time making love than cohabitating or dating couples.

A long-term partner who really supports your work and goals is sexy.

There are many advantages to monogamous sex, and it can be a lot of fun.

A good sex life makes a marriage a love affair.

I've learned that...

Remaining seductive—flirting, dressing up, nibbling his neck, leaving her love notes—is part of a successful long-term relationship.

An older couple dancing alone on the dance floor makes everyone watching feel good.

Every long-term relationship involves disappointments; people who don't try to change each other are happier.

A lifelong partner usually does not have all the characteristics of your idealized fantasy lover.

There really is a honeymoon effect: sexual frequency DOES go down after the first year of marriage.

The biggest enemy of sex in long-term relationships is anger.

The partner with lower desire always controls the sexual relationship.

I've learned that...

The most common reason people give for not having sex in a long-term relationship is fatigue; but sometimes people are tired because they are bored.

The quality of the relationship is almost always determined by both partners.

Less than a third of married couples say they have taken a shower together.

In order not to get bored, couples need to vary their routine in bed.

Our society makes it seem like lifelong marriage is almost impossible to achieve.

A good long-term relationship includes trust: continuing jealousy means something is wrong.

It is very hard to break out of sexual ruts in a long-term relationship.

I've learned that...

It's easy to think that you know your partner's body and desires perfectly—and upsetting to find out you do not. And this is even truer about their thoughts.

One secret to renewing your belief in your relationship is to go over a scrapbook full of wonderful memories.

This works best when you are feeling good about your relationship. When you're worried about your marriage, you tend to only remember what went wrong on that vacation or holiday.

Partners must continue to work at being attractive in long-term relationships.

More than eight in ten married couples say they are physically and emotionally pleased with their sex lives.

15

About
MASTURBATION

I've learned that...

Most highly sexual people masturbate a lot.

Few people are comfortable talking about their own experiences with masturbation.

Sometimes I want to masturbate frequently . . . and sometimes I go for weeks without it.

People in happy sexual relationships still masturbate.

It is normal to masturbate, and it is normal not to.

I've learned that...

Watching a partner masturbate can be exciting.

Mutual masturbation is a great way to have sex without taking any risks.

Some women can't have an orgasm with new partners until they have masturbated in front of them.

Masturbation techniques are highly individual.

You can't teach another person to masturbate; they need to experiment by themselves.

Sometimes I masturbate for pleasure, and sometimes I do so just to relieve stress.

Sometimes I masturbate to orgasm in less than two minutes, and sometimes I make love to myself for hours.

Most married or cohabitating people don't tell their partners when they masturbate.

Many women have stronger orgasms when they masturbate than when they have sex with a partner.

I've learned that...

Attitudes about masturbation change very slowly.

There is no such thing as too much masturbation, unless it is interfering with your life, relationship, or work.

Most teenagers deny masturbating.

More men than women masturbate.

Masturbation is a great way to learn about what excites you.

Married people masturbate more than single people.

Studies report that 60 percent of men and 40 percent of women masturbate—and I think the numbers are actually higher.

Masturbating to orgasm helps menstrual cramps.

People develop a particular highly individual way to masturbate to climax.

I like to carry a small vibrator with me when I travel.

$\mathcal{I}$'ve learned that...

You can buy a vibrator in almost any drugstore; it's usually marketed as a back massager.

If you want a fancy vibrator, you'll find one in a mail-order catalog. I found mine listed in an ad in the Sunday *New York Times* book section.

Most people find one sexual fantasy to masturbate with and use it over and over again—especially when they are close to orgasm.

People still worry about whether they are masturbating too much.

Once is too much if you don't like it.

Many men and women do not need erotic materials to masturbate.

Some women can have an orgasm just riding in a vibrating train, bus, or car . . . and they love that no one around them knows.

16

About
PEAK EVENTS

I've learned that...
You never forget your peak experiences.

For some people, passionate kissing and fondling in public are some of the most arousing ways they can turn each other on, but they may turn off the people around them.

A lot of people belong to the "mile high club" and consider making love in an airplane a peak event in their sexual life together.

Whenever people do something "kinky" for the first time, it is either a peak event or an awful failure.

I've learned that...

For most people the wedding night is not a peak sexual event.

Having sex with the person you've always wanted to have sex with is not usually the peak event you thought it would be.

The best sex happens when you feel totally accepted as a person.

A peak experience takes place when we are truly one and merge both flesh and soul.

Sex with just the right amount of champagne can be a peak experience.

There are lots of wonderful uses for champagne during sex.

There's nothing sexier than a candlelit bathroom, great-smelling bath bubbles and a tub that's large enough for two.

I've learned that. . .

You don't have to be with someone you love to have a peak sexual experience (they don't even have to speak your language).

Everyone deserves one "Bridges of Madison County" weekend.

Making love in risky places often produces amazing sex because the heightened sense of desire overwhelms wisdom or restraint.

When you decide together that a certain night will be the start of making a baby, it can be a peak sexual experience.

The first time is rarely a peak physical experience, but you never forget it.

In a long-term relationship you usually have to plan new peak experiences.

A really luxurious hotel room can go a long way in setting the stage for a peak sexual experience.

I've learned that...

Peak experiences can happen almost anywhere—on the beach, in the woods, even in your own bed.

For some people, a peak experience is a sacred experience.

Sex after almost breaking up can be a peak event.

I use my peak events over and over again as fantasy material.

You shouldn't try to repeat a specific peak event.

Peak experiences don't happen very often.

Peak events don't have to be spontaneous.

You can use contraceptives and condoms during a peak event.

Some peak events do not include intercourse.

Sex in the movies almost always looks like a peak event.

The movies can give you good scenarios for peak events.

What I've Learned About Sex

I've learned that...

It's hard to share my peak events with my girlfriends—it's too personal or embarrassing.

Not every marriage needs peak events.

Most peak events are shared by both partners.

Sometimes only one of you is having a peak event.

You can gain useful information if you ask your partner, "What do you think was the best sex we've ever had?"

17

About
PLEASURE

I've learned that...

You have to know how to pleasure yourself before you can be a good lover to someone else.

Orgasm doesn't have to be the goal of sex. Sometimes the excitement is more than enough.

For all-night winter delight, sleep in the nude on flannel sheets.

The eyes are the most erotic part of the body; being "touched" by someone's eyes can be an incredible turn-on.

I've learned that. . .

It's just as important to receive as to give. Someone who can't receive denies their partner the pleasure of giving.

Orgasm varies depending on the time of the month, the partner, the mood—and all the variations can be pleasurable.

Sex is better when my partner and I are equally matched in passion, creativity, and desire for intimacy.

Women reach orgasms via different paths, through clitoral stimulation, vaginal stimulation, cervical stimulation, and breast stimulation. For a few women, imagery alone leads to orgasm, without anyone, including the woman herself, touching her body.

The best sex happens when you are both concentrating more on each other's pleasure than on your own.

Most people concentrate on their own pleasure.

Quickies are usually better for men than for women.

I've learned that...

It's the rare man who truly devotes himself to a woman's pleasures.

Some men report they have multiple orgasms—but I haven't met any.

Some women swear that they have a G spot; and some women swear they don't.

Vibrators do wonders for some women . . . and are way too intense for others.

When I am really turned on, every part of my body becomes an erogenous zone.

Some women feel sexiest at midcycle, some during their periods, some immediately after. Every woman should pay attention to her own cycles.

There are few really gifted lovers.

The average married couple makes love 57 times a year . . . that's once a week and three times on vacation.

I've learned that...

For most couples, vaginal intercourse lasts fewer minutes than it takes for women to come through intercourse alone.

I need to trust my feelings during sex; if it feels good, I let myself enjoy it.

If you tell people what you like, they just may do it.

Most men don't know if women are faking.

Most men say that they always have an orgasm during sex, but only one in three women say that they do. Unfortunately, many more men than women report that their partners climax all the time.

Women who generally fake orgasms with their partners are cheating themselves.

Men don't just perform oral sex for their partners' pleasure. In one large national study, 90 percent of men said that they enjoyed performing oral sex.

I've learned that...

The biggest enemies of pleasure are anxiety, anger, and guilt.

Sometimes parts of my body that aren't ordinarily aroused can surprise me and suddenly feel exquisite when touched.

Verbal sounds of my partner's pleasure add immeasurably to my excitement.

I can't always predict how pleasurable any given night of lovemaking will be.

One of the greatest pleasures in the world is anticipation.

The line between pleasurable stroking and tickling is dangerously close.

People are responsible for their own sexual pleasure.

18

About
RAISING
SEXUALLY HEALTHY
CHILDREN

I've learned that...

It's parents' responsibility to teach values about sexuality to their children.

Both moms and dads have this responsibility.

Sex education begins in the delivery room when you ask "Is it a boy or a girl?"

Boy babies need as much cuddling and verbal interaction as girl babies.

Even small children understand what it is to be masculine and feminine.

I've learned that...

I need to teach my children all the parts of their bodies; it's not okay to say, "This is your nose, this is your belly, these are your knees" and ignore a third of the body.

Parents can start off using the words "penis" and "vulva," not "down there" or cute names.

All babies like to touch their genitals.

A parent's reaction to this gives the child a strong message about sexuality.

Three-year-olds ask questions about sex at the most inopportune times—in line at the supermarket, in church, in front of the in-laws.

By age 3 at the latest, children have a clear sense of gender identification: they know if they are a boy or a girl.

By age 4, a child will ask, "Where do babies come from?" and parents should rehearse their answers.

Age 3 is not too early to teach your child about privacy.

I've learned that. . .

Most parents are embarrassed talking to their children about sexuality. You don't have to be comfortable to do a good job.

There is help for parents on how to talk about sex; books, courses, and agencies can help you.

Preschoolers like to "play doctor." Think ahead about what you will do if you find your children and the neighbors' kids without their clothes on.

It's better not to place adult meanings on child sexual play.

I look for "teachable moments" with my child—a pregnant friend is a good way to introduce a fact of life.

I should not wait for my children to ask questions about sex.

It's important to give very simple answers to small children.

If I give too much information, they just stop listening.

I've learned that...

Once children start kindergarten, they start learning about sexual issues from their friends and classmates.

Today's 6-year-olds have heard about AIDS, gay people, intercourse, and other adult topics, and that's why it's hard to ignore these subjects.

Even early elementary students have boyfriends and girl-friends.

Some girls start menstruating by the age of 8; all girls need to know about periods by then.

Girls start to care about what their bodies look like by fifth grade. Low self-esteem about body image can lead to eating disorders.

Both boys and girls need to learn about the changes of puberty by age 8 or 9.

Some people celebrate their daughter's first period and make the experience really special.

I've learned that. . .

"The big talk" about sex never works. It just embarrasses both of you. Educating your children about sexuality is a gradual, ongoing process.

If parents haven't been open with their children about sexuality until puberty, their preteens are unlikely to be open with them.

As children enter adolescence, they may no longer feel comfortable talking to their own parents about sex—even if the parents are sexuality educators. Make sure they have another trustworthy adult to talk to about sexuality.

Most middle-school kids don't date, but they do start to "go with people." This mainly means that they can announce that somebody "likes them."

Parents CAN set limits on dating, makeup, and dress—even if they're contrary to what's "cool."

Forty percent of ninth graders have had intercourse at least once, and it's not safe to assume that it is always someone else's ninth-grade child.

I've learned that...

The time to start talking with my kids about setting sexual limits and birth control is before they start to date.

If your teenager is in love and spending time alone with their beloved, there's a good chance they may be having intercourse.

Parents should stay involved in their teenagers' lives and ask questions.

It's critical to tell my children if I think they are too young to have intercourse but it's also vital that they know how to protect themselves.

If I think my teenage children might be sexually active, both my daughter and my son need to know how to get and use condoms.

Offering to take your son or daughter to get contraception can help them protect themselves . . . and let them know you're really there for them.

I've learned that...

Parents don't have to answer the question "How old were you when you first had sex?"

Teens need parents' support for saying "no."

Even for sexologists, it's emotionally difficult to accept that your teenager is having sex.

19

About
SAYING "NO"

I've learned that...

Adults do go through periods of abstinence.

It's better to set sexual limits—and agree to stick to them—before any sexual behaviors begin.

There are an infinite number of safe and very sexy behaviors that do not involve intercourse.

I miss just making out for hours at a time.

Only 3 percent of American adults are virgins.

$\mathcal{I}$'ve learned that...

A professional massage can be all the touching I need when I am not having sex with a partner.

I prefer abstinence to having sex with people I don't care about.

There are many ways to say "no" without hurting the other person's feelings.

The more secure a person is, the easier it is to say—or accept—"no."

Saying "Not tonight, dear" is not a big deal in a good relationship, but a problem when a couple is not getting along.

You can only say "no" to your partner a few times in a row; after that it feels like rejection.

It's easier for me to say "no" than to hear it from my partner.

Men need permission to say "no" too.

I've learned that...

Masturbating helps get one through a period of abstinence.

Ejaculating after a period of abstinence feels especially intense.

Almost half of single women and single men had little or no sex during the past year.

Sex is really not important to some people.

It's a myth that it's easy for women to find sex partners.

Saying "no" feels very powerful.

Movies and television shows don't offer examples of how to say "no" and still have a happy ending.

People cannot believe an abstinent person is a happy person.

Abstinence can be a relief after a bad marriage or a failed love affair.

What I've Learned About Sex

I've learned that...

A lot of men still believe that when a woman says "no" she just wants to be convinced and "swept away."

Some men don't care whether or not a woman says "no"; today, those men may be successfully prosecuted.

Sometimes it's the woman who doesn't want to take "no" for an answer.

Teaching teenagers ONLY about abstinence is not enough.

Vows of abstinence are hard to keep; they fail more than condoms do.

Abstinence doesn't make the heart grow fonder.

People leaving a long-term relationship are afraid that they will never have another sexual partner.

If I am not sure about saying "yes," I should say "no."

It's better not to say "yes" just to be nice. My feelings are as important as those of the person asking.

I've learned that...

There are 35-year-old virgins.

There are married couples who don't have sex at all.

A lot of women wish they had said "no" more often.

Sometimes men are relieved when a woman says "no."

I don't like it . . . abstinence, that is.

About
SEX
AFTER 40

I've learned that...
You can have fulfilling sex-
ual experiences at 90, if you're healthy and sexually
involved at 60, 70, and 80.

Older men usually need to have their penises
touched before they get an erection. It's not personal—it's physical.

Older women usually lubricate less.

A good lover after 40 is a patient lover.

You need different information about sex after 40;
it's not like having sex at 18.

I've learned that...

Elderly people still masturbate.

Sex improves with intimacy and age.

A 49-year-old woman can still attract 25-year-olds.

A rich and powerful 80-year-old man can still attract some 25-year-olds.

Many women are more sexually self-confident after 40, and their self-confidence makes them better lovers.

Men and women have a more subtle sexuality as they age.

It is not necessarily a bad thing that older men take longer to come—in fact, it's a good thing.

I worry about whether I will still be sexually attractive as I age.

Menopause affects many women's sexuality; some women feel stronger, more powerful and sexier, while others find that their sexual interest declines.

You can have great sex with a soft penis.

$\mathcal{I}$'ve learned that...

Older women should discuss using testosterone with their physician if their sexual drive is decreasing.

The changes associated with menopause can begin as many as ten years before periods cease.

Some people have problems finding sexual partners as they get older, but really sexually alive people don't seem to have this difficulty.

Our culture makes fun of people over 65 who are still sexually interested and involved, and that hurts all of us.

People who didn't like sex much when they were younger tend to give it up after age 50.

Men ejaculate with less force as they get older.

Many older people take medicines that can negatively affect their sexual desire.

People can have fulfilling, active sex lives after they've had a heart attack without risking their health. It's no more dangerous than climbing a flight of stairs—and a lot more fun.

I've learned that...

The riskiest sex after a heart attack is with someone be-sides your spouse.

Even though a young person may consider an older person asexual, they are rarely correct.

Physically fit older people stay interested in sex longer.

If an older partner loses interest in sex, it may be a sign of depression.

People will have a variety of reactions to an older woman who dresses seductively.

I should not dress too young for my age.

The older I get, the farther away the age one becomes elderly gets.

People who were really attractive in their youth may not be willing to admit that they are aging.

There really is such a thing as too many face-lifts.

Some men and women are sexy forever. Cases in point: Greta Garbo, Clark Gable, and Mae West.

I've learned that...

As many men get older, they become more interested in cuddling and caressing—and that's good news.

Having sex with someone younger than you are can make you feel younger too.

Having sex when you are older can make you feel younger.

For more
INFORMATION
About SEXUALITY . . .
Contact the Following
ORGANIZATIONS:

American Association of Sex Educators, Counselors, and Therapists
PO Box 238
Mt. Vernon, IA 52314
319-895-8407
This organization will provide you with a list of certified sex counselors and therapists in your area.

Sexuality Information and Education Council of the United States
130 W. 42nd Street
Suite 350
New York, NY 10036
212-819-9770
http://www.siecus.org
This group is an excellent resource for general information about sexuality.

Society for the Scientific Study of Sexuality
PO Box 208
Mt. Vernon, IA 52314
319-895-8407
Contact this organization for research about sexuality.

Hotlines and 800 Numbers

Bisexual Resource Center
617-424-9595

Domestic Violence Hotline
1-800-799-SAFE

Emergency Contraception Hotline
1-800-584-9911

**Information Center for Individuals
with Disabilities**
1-800-462-5015

National Abortion Federation
1-800-772-9100

National AIDS Hotline
English 1-800-342-AIDS
Spanish 1-800-344-7432
TTY 1-800-243-7889

National Gay and Lesbian Task Force
202-332-6483

National Genetics Foundation
212-586-5800

National Health Information Clearinghouse
1-800-336-4797

National Institute on Aging Information Center
1-800-222-2225

National STD Hotline
1-800-227-8922

PMS/Menopause Hotline
1-800-222-4767

Planned Parenthood Federation of America
1-800-829-PPFA

What I've Learned About Sex

Internet Addresses

This list of Internet addresses was compiled by the staff from the Sexuality Information and Education Council of the United States during the summer of 1996. You may want to use a search engine to find information on a specific topic. This list is not intended as an endorsement, as content changes rapidly on the Internet. As any net user knows, the quality of information on the net is highly variable, and users need to beware.

The **SIECUS** Web site provides general information on topics relating to sexuality: http://www.siecus.org

The **Kinsey Institute** Web site has good research information: http://www.indiana.edu/kinsey

Planned Parenthood Federation of America provides a Web site on contraception that includes a listing of clinic locations: http://www.ppfa.org/ppfa

The American Social Health Association has a Web site that deals primarily with STDs: http://sunsite.unc.edu/asha

Columbia University's Web site on sexuality issues addresses young adults and their questions: http://www.columbia.edu/cu/healthwise

The U.S. Centers for Disease Control (CDC) National AIDS Clearinghouse provides up-to-date AIDS information on their Web site: http://www.cdcnac.org

WHAT HAVE YOU LEARNED ABOUT SEX? We would like to hear from you for possible future books. Send your one-line statements to:

Debra W. Haffner MPH and Pepper Schwartz, Ph.D.
c/o Perigee Books
375 Hudson Street
New York, NY 10014

We will list you in an acknowledgments section, but will not attribute your statement by name.